Survivor's Guide to Chemo 2.0

Dr. Deborah Waun

DEDICATION

This book is dedicated to my wonderful mother (Alison Waun) who spent her entire life helping others (as a mother, a pastor's wife, a caseworker for social services, and a DAR member helping the community). She has set an example for other Christian women to follow. God gave me one of the greatest blessings there is by allowing me to have her as my mother. She sacrificed things for herself so she could give more time; she sacrificed time for herself by working to help provide for me, and then gave me whatever leisure time she had; and she continued to give of herself in order to give me a better life right up until she was bedridden. I am here today because my loving mother nursed me back to health, went with me to every doctor's appointment and chemo treatment, and encouraged me every step of the way.

CONTENTS

Acknowledgments

Introduction   1

My Story   5

1   Treatment Plan & Side Effects   29

2   CA-125   34

3   Side Effects of Chemo   36

4   Do NOT Eat Popcorn!   40

5   Food   43

6   Loss of Appetite   50

7   Nausea   54

8   Hygiene   57

9   Hair   62

10   White Blood Cells   66

11   Depression   70

12   Keep a Positive Attitude   76

13   Support Groups   80

14   24-Hour Emergency Hotline   82

15   Getting a Port   84

16	Antibiotics	93
17	Accept Help	95
18	Financial Assistance	97
	Corresponding Therapies	100
	Ovarian Cancer Info	107
	Symptoms	112
	New Research	114
	Authors Note	120
	References	121
	About the Author	123

ACKNOWLEDGMENTS

Special Thanks

To my heroes: Dr. John L. Powell and Dr. Adnan Taj-Eldin for saving my life.

To my best friends: Mary Hughes and Laurel Schaefer for their prayers, cards, phone calls and encouragement.

To my brother: the Rev. Dr. William G. Waun for coming to my rescue whenever I needed him.

To all the nurses at the Zimmer Center and New Hanover Regional Medical Center who helped me through surgery and chemo treatments.

And to all my friends and family who prayed for me, emailed me, sent flowers and cards, and called to support me.

SURVIVOR'S GUIDE TO CHEMO 2.0

FORWARD

I have been treating women with ovarian cancer for over thirty years. Many changes have occurred in that time period in surgical techniques, new chemotherapy drugs, anti-emetics, and bone-marrow stimulating medicines. Throughout those years, I have always been amazed by and admired the courage, strength, determination to survive and endure, gratitude, and kindness of my patients. Deborah Waun's book will be a helpful guide with useful tips, and inspiration to other women facing the challenge of ovarian cancer.

The fortunate person, in my opinion, is he/she to whom the gods have granted the power either to do something which is worth recording or to write what is worth reading, and most fortunate of all is the person who can do both.

John L. Powell, M.D., FACOG, FACS
Director, Gynecologic Oncology
New Hanover Regional Medical Center
Southeastern Area Health Education Center
Professor Obstetrics and Gynecology
University of North Carolina School of Medicine

INTRODUCTION

I wrote this handbook in order to help those going through chemotherapy. I began taking notes during the time that I was undergoing chemo treatments so that I could pass along all of the information that I was learning through my own experience. I hope that these ideas and tips will help you get through your experience with as little pain and discomfort at possible.

In this book, I have included brand name products to have on hand and specific things that you can do to help relieve pain. This book is compiled in a way that is conducive to someone who does not feel well and just wants to go right to the information that they need. Often when one does not feel well, they may not feel like reading and searching through a book to find what will help them. This handbook is short and to-the-point, and easy to read. The purpose of this information is to empower you as you embark upon your own journey to wellness. Knowledge is power.

First, you should understand how urgent and life-threatening ovarian cancer is. According to Kunle Odunsi, M.D., Ph.D. (2018), "Ovarian cancer often progresses significantly before a patient is diagnosed. This is because the symptoms of ovarian cancer can be easily confused with less life-threatening digestive issues such as bloating, constipation, and gas. Roughly only 20 percent of ovarian cancers are detected before it spreads beyond the ovaries. The most prominent risk factor for this disease is a family history that includes breast or ovarian cancer. Women who test positive for the inherited mutations in the BRCA1 or BRCA2 genes are at significantly greater risk—45% to 65% risk of developing breast cancer and

10% to 20% risk of developing ovarian cancer by age 70. Women at age 40 are at the highest risk" (para. 1).

Odunsi (2018) goes on to say that, "Globally, ovarian cancer is diagnosed in an estimated 300,000 women each year and causes roughly 180,000 deaths. In 2018, ovarian cancer was diagnosed in approximately 22,000 women and caused about 14,000 deaths in the United States, where it is the leading cause of death from gynecologic cancer. While significant advances have been made in surgical and chemo-based treatments for ovarian cancer, the survival rates have only modestly improved. The poor survival in advanced ovarian cancer is due both to late diagnosis as well as to the lack of effective second-line therapy for patients who relapse. Many women affected by advanced ovarian cancer respond to chemotherapy, but effects are not typically long-lasting. The clinical course of ovarian cancer patients is marked by periods of remission and relapse of sequentially shortening duration until chemotherapy resistance develops. More than 80% of ovarian cancer patients experience recurrent disease, and more than 50% of these patients die from the disease in less than five years post-diagnosis" (para. 3).

These facts are the reason why my doctor proclaimed that I am a miracle! I was sick for several months and had numerous symptoms many months prior to that, and I had a basketball-sized tumor. I beat the odds, but I attribute that to all of the prayers lifted up for me. God is certainly my shield and my protector! "The LORD is my rock, my fortress, and my savior; my God is my rock, in whom I find protection. He is my shield, the power that saves me, and my place of safety." Psalm 18:2.

MY STORY

When hearing the diagnosis of "you have cancer," everyone probably has the same reaction… "No, not me!" I was 48 and had been very healthy all of my life, so the idea of cancer seemed absurd!

I grew up in a small town in Indiana. My father was a minister, my mother was a social worker, and I was the baby and only girl in my family with two older brothers. After graduating from college and a brief marriage, I moved to Los Angeles and worked in the entertainment industry for 14 years. In 2000, I moved to Atlanta to help take care of my dad who had been diagnosed with a rare incurable illness. I helped my mom care for him for the last six months of his life. At the time, I believed that taking care of my dad and seeing him in pain would be the hardest thing I ever would do, but life is not always what we expect it to be.

I enjoyed living in California and especially loved my job in casting. It was fun being able to find the right actor for the television role. However, casting, as with any job, can be very stressful at times. The biggest take away from this book is that stress breaks down the immune system. So, if you have a lot of stress in your life, you need to find ways to relieve it.

I grew up in a Christian home with loving parents who did everything to enable me to have a good life. My parents sacrificed many things in order to provide for their children, so when my dad got sick, I knew it was time to make some changes in my life and help him. I quit my job in casting and moved to Atlanta to live with my parents and help care for my dad. This was a very difficult time because I watched my big strong father deteriorate and become weak and helpless.

My dad had dedicated his life to serving the

Lord and helping to lead others to Christ. My dad was a leader and a take-charge kind of man. He had a vision and worked hard to achieve it. But his illness got stronger and made him weaker and weaker. There were many times that he would fall and couldn't get up, which progressed to him not being able to get out of bed. It doesn't matter how old you are, when your dad can no longer be your protector, your security disappears.

On December 16, 2001, I was with him when he passed away. Even though I was in my 40's, I felt like a little girl when I lost him. It was during that time that I decided I wanted to help people who were going through rough times. While working full-time, I pursued my Masters' degree in Psychology and became a Licensed Professional Counselor.

For the next few years my mother and I lived together in Atlanta while I completed the required supervision for licensure. In the meantime, my brother and his family moved to North Carolina. I realized how difficult it was to take care of my dad and knew that I would probably need help caring for my mom as she got older, so I suggested that we move to be near my brother.

I cannot pinpoint the exact time that I started getting sick. Looking back on it now, I believe it was during the stressful time that I was caring for my dad. I did not take care of myself during that time. I worked full-time and then would come home and start taking care of my dad in order to relieve my mom. I would force myself to be positive and upbeat around my parents but at night when I would go to bed, I would cry myself to sleep. Also, my parents were old-school and believed that you don't pay for things that you can do yourself. So, I ended up being the lawncare service, house cleaner, shopper, etc. I realize now that I should have paid to have some of those things done but I was the dutiful daughter.

Deciding to move, added another layer of work to my list. My mother was 80 so I did most of the packing. I also contacted realtors, researched new homes in North Carolina, dealt with the financial advisor, screened moving companies, and continued packing. When the movers came, I helped them carry things to the moving van, I cleaned the house and helped with staging it for open houses. Once the house sold, I packed the car and drove 9 hours to our new home. Upon arrival, I helped the movers unload the van. I went through all of the boxes in the garage which was stacked full, I unpacked, moved furniture, moved heavy boxes to areas for unpacking, all in July with temperatures of 90 – 100 degrees. I never stopped going, until I collapsed!

While unpacking and organizing furniture, I was also filling out insurance paperwork for damaged property from the move, working on getting my counseling license in North Carolina, and looking for a job. My brother warned me to slow down and take a break, but that wasn't me. I guess they didn't realize that I was superwoman! I say this with tongue-in-cheek because nobody can be superwoman. Something has to give. All that stress was weakening my immune system.

I noticed that I was fatigued and would fall asleep while sitting in a chair in the early evening. That was unusual for me because I always need quiet and darkness in order to sleep. In mid-August, my stomach started hurting and I began to feel nauseated. I realized that I couldn't burp or pass gas. My stomach and abdomen began bloating and I had a fever. The fever started at 103 degrees for one night and then if ranged between 99 and 101. My stomach began cramping and I lost my appetite. I started feeling sick all of the time and it became painful to eat or even drink water.

As I reflect, I realize that I had other symptoms that I had chalked up to getting older. Five months prior to getting really sick, my abdomen started to bloat, and I had acid reflux when I went to bed. I was also on edge and irritable much of the time. And I had to urinate more frequently.

We had only been in North Carolina for a month, so I did not have a doctor yet. Since I did not have a doctor, I went to the Urgent Care where I was examined, and blood and urine tests were taken. The tests did not indicate any problem and my white blood cell count was not elevated so I believed that whatever the problem was, at least it couldn't be cancer because when you have cancer, your white blood cells elevate so they can fight off the infection. I was wrong! The Urgent Care doctor diagnosed me with gastroenteritis, suggested that I see a Gastroenterologist, prescribed an elixir (Belladonna®) to help with stomach cramps, and sent me on my way.

I immediately made an appointment with a Gastroenterologist, but his first opening was not until October 12th and this was mid-August. There are only two Gastroenterologists in the town where I lived, and they were both booked solid until Mid-October. I am usually a proactive person but when you are sick and new to an area, you feel helpless.

Things continued to get worse. My symptoms grew to include diarrhea. As previously mentioned, I had already lost my appetite and my stomach hurt whenever I ate or drank. I felt sick all of the time and I began losing weight. Since I was getting worse, I went to the emergency room at the local hospital. I waited for six hours before I was seen by a doctor. He examined me, took more blood and urine, and an x-ray. All of the tests came back clean because they were not testing for cancer. I made the mistake of telling him the diagnosis that the urgent care doctor had given me. If you are ever in the situation where you are getting a second opinion, don't tell them what the first doctor said because it is too easy for the next doctor to just accept that diagnosis. And that is exactly what happened.

I went home to continue waiting for six long weeks for my appointment with the Gastroenterologist. I was so sick. It is hard to describe exactly how I felt. I had a fever, had constant stomach pain, was bloated and couldn't pass gas, was fatigued, had diarrhea, and was depressed. Since I was always in pain, I couldn't sleep. This continued to worsen in the next 45 days.

I was desperate to find out what was happening to me. I researched the internet searching to find out what I had. I thought that maybe I had a parasite since some of the symptoms were similar, so I went back to Urgent Care and asked them to test for that.

While I was at Urgent Care, the doctor told me that he could get me in with a local MD. I was able to get an appointment in the next few days and finally I was going to get a definitive answer. Dr. Eldin had a practice in the same neighborhood where I lived. He examined me and felt a tumor. In his words, he said he felt a "very large tumor!"

Two days later on September 25th I had a CT scan which revealed a huge tumor in my abdomen. This information was immediately given to Dr. Eldin who called me into his office right away. He explained to me that I had a "basketball sized" tumor which he believed was most likely ovarian cancer. He suggested that I see a cancer specialist at the Zimmer Cancer Center in Wilmington (1 ½ hours away). When giving referrals, most doctors hand the patient a card with the referral number on it and let them make the call. However, Dr. Eldin knew how urgent this was so he made the call himself.

When Dr. Eldin left the room to call the specialist, I prayed that God would help me, and that the specialist would be able to see me right away. After the call, Dr. Eldin came back in to tell me that the specialist would see me the next day at 9:00 a.m. What are the chances that a busy well-known cancer specialist, (Dr. John L. Powell) would be available to see me first thing the next day? As it turned out, Dr. Powell is not only well-known, but he is one of the nation's leading gynecological oncologists.

My brother (the Rev. Dr. William G. Waun) dropped everything on his busy schedule to drive my mother and me to Wilmington. Dr. Eldin had suggested that I take an overnight bag with me on the off-chance that they would admit me to the hospital. I also took the CT scan with me.

Dr. John Powell met with all three of us, looked at the CT scan and didn't pull any punches. He told me directly that I had ovarian cancer. He said that I needed surgery including a complete hysterectomy, and removal of other body parts such as my gall bladder, appendix, and lymph nodes. This was such a shock to me! I just couldn't believe that I had cancer! I questioned Dr. Powell and asked about the possibility that the tumor was benign. He replied that it most certainly was *not* benign.

My head was reeling, and I didn't even know what questions to ask. It is always a good idea to take someone with you in situations like this because your emotions make it difficult to concentrate and think clearly. My brother asked what my prognosis was, and Dr. Powell replied that he would not know until he opened me up in surgery. But he said one thing he could tell us is that this cancer was fast-growing and aggressive.

I was then ushered into another room where

I was examined, and several vials of blood were drawn. The realization of everything was setting in and a wave of fear and sorrow overwhelmed me. I was worried that I might not survive the surgery. One of the nurses (Nicole) came in to comfort me and reassure me. Even though I was scared, I desperately wanted to get the tumor out of me! I was concerned that I might have to wait for several days before Dr. Powell would have time to perform my surgery. As I sat there alone waiting for Dr. Powell to return, I started praying that God would work it out so that I could have the surgery right away. When Dr. Powell came in, he told me that he would be performing my surgery at noon the next day. I believe that this was another answer to prayer.

The next step was to be admitted to New Hanover Regional Medical Center which is adjacent to the Zimmer Center. My mother and brother accompanied me to my hospital room and helped me settle in for the night, and then they headed back home. That's when the fear really set in! As I sat there all alone in the hospital room, the realization of everything began to sink in. I called my friends to say my good byes just in case.

As I was laying in the hospital bed, the worst-case scenarios kept creeping into my head, and I began to cry. I started praying and asking God to help me. While I was praying the sweetest nurse (Shirley) came in and asked me what she could do to make me feel better. I asked her if she would pray for me and she did not hesitate. She hugged me and took my hand and began to pray. Then she sat with me and reassured me that everything would be okay. She was there when I needed someone. Nurses give totally of themselves and I was fortunate to have some of the best take care of me.

The next morning before the surgery, (thanks to Shirley), several nurses and a doctor came into my room and formed a circle around me along with my mother, brother, and sister-in-law, and they all prayed for me. This kind of care and concern is what makes a hospital stand out. Before I knew it, they were wheeling me down the hall for the surgery. As you are being wheeled on a stretcher to have major surgery, there is a real feeling of how alone you are. Your family can't be with you. It is just you and God.

My family was taken to a waiting room and I was taken to pre-op where I met the Assisting Doctor, the Anesthesiologist, and the Operating Room Nurse whose name was Ruth. Ruth was very kind and promised that she would watch over me during the surgery. The last thing that I remember is being offered a shot for pain. I don't even remember receiving the shot. And as if no time had passed, I woke up in my hospital room with a large tube down my throat which prevented me from speaking. And of course, nobody was in my room!

It wasn't long before a nurse came in and noticed that I was awake and shortly after that Dr. Powell came to see me. The surgery had included a complete hysterectomy and removal of some of my lymph nodes. Dr. Powell said that he usually removes certain organs during surgery because he knows where the cancer cells like to hide. He had planned to remove other organs but when he opened me up, he was surprised to see that the cancer was contained in the tumor! When you think about how long I had been sick, how large the tumor was, and the fact that ovarian cancer usually spreads throughout the body very quickly, it is a miracle that I am alive!

Dr. Powell said that I was in Stage One (the best stage) and he believed that he removed all of the cancer. He also said that all of my organs looked clean. I think that he was amazed that I was not filled with cancer. I later found out that I was in surgery much longer than what was anticipated because the extremely large tumor was wrapped around organs and muscles. I had to be given a transfusion because I lost so much blood. But God spared my life! Prayer still works!

Even though Dr. Powell believed he had

removed all of the cancer, he still suggested that I receive chemotherapy. He let me know that cancer cells can hide and there was still the possibility that some may be lurking inside of me. He said if I elected to get chemo, he wanted to wait for a month in order to give my body time to heal and build up some strength.

I will always consider Dr. Powell to be my hero because he saved my life. Webster's dictionary defines hero as, "One distinguished for action, a brave man, noble, conqueror, champion, man of great courage, a man among men." I submit that doctors who dedicate themselves to trying to save lives and go into battle daily against disease are heroes. This goes for nurses too. They have to face people everyday with bad news and sometimes watch them get worse while they do their best to fight their illnesses. I couldn't help myself, but my hero stepped in and saved me. I can't think of anyone who better fits the definition of hero than Dr. Powell.

I was fortunate to have a private room and wonderful nurses. Since visiting hours were over by the time that I awoke, my family had left, but I wasn't alone for long. I had caring nurses checking on me all night. I also had several phone calls from friends and family. Three things that I advise anyone to take if they are having an overnight stay at the hospital are earplugs, a neck pillow, and an eye mask. These three items will help you be able to sleep in a place that stays active at all hours.

I was in the hospital for seven days after the surgery and I was on a liquid diet most of that time. They switched me to solid food the morning that I was to be released with the condition that I had to eat solid food before I could leave. The problem was that food repulsed me. And they brought in bacon, eggs and a biscuit. This would not be what I would suggest for a first meal after not eating for a week. I wanted to go home so I nibbled on the biscuit, covered up the other food, and told them that I ate my breakfast. I guess nobody checked because they allowed me to leave!

On October 3rd I finally got to go home! I was very weak and still felt sick but there's no place like home! My brother and mother came to get me and helped me settle in to the backseat of his minivan for the 1 ½ hour ride home. My mom brought a blanket for me which was a good idea since it was a while before I could get my body temperature regulated and I was always cold.

Prior to leaving the hospital, I was told that I could eat anything that I wanted. It would have been nice if they would have given me a list of food that one should not eat when recovering from surgery because I chose one of the worst things to eat after I got home. I thought that eating a few bites of banana would be good but as I later found out, banana is very hard to digest. And I found out the hard way! It hit me around midnight and lasted for several hours. The pain was terrible! It felt like my stomach and intestines were on fire. All that I could do was stand and pace while holding my stomach and crying. I did not realize that it was the banana making me sick and I was worried that something serious was wrong.

The next day the pain had eased but I still felt sick, so I called the doctor's office and spoke to his nurse (Debbie) who told me that it was most likely the banana. She suggested that I take some Maalox to soothe my stomach and it really helped. She also asked the doctor to prescribe some medication (Aciphex®) which helps break down the acid in the stomach. In addition, she suggested that I try eating Jell-O, popsicles, or pudding along with drinking Special K water, Pedialyte, or Gatorade. These are all foods/fluids that are easy to digest along with helping to keep you hydrated and providing nutrients. I called Debbie several times with questions while I was recuperating, and she was always very kind and helpful.

In case you are not aware, you do not need to get your prescriptions fully filled. You can get them half-filled until you see if you need more. I spent a lot of money getting a pain medication (Oxycodone®) filled, only to find out that I didn't need it.

I experienced pain in my shoulders, upper
back and sides which I believe was trapped gas.
My mother suggested putting heat on the areas that
hurt and much to my surprise the pain went away.
Every time I had that type of pain, I heated up a
little microwavable bean bag and held it to the area
and the pain would dissipate.

On October 8th (5 days after being released
from the hospital and 11 days after surgery) I had
my staples removed. Since the tumor had been so
large, I had to have an incision that was also very
large, and that incision was held together by several
very large staples! The doctor removed the staples
with what looks like a very large staple remover. It
was at this appointment that Dr. Powell gave me
more information about getting chemo.

My sister-in-law (Cynthia) did some
research for me so I would be better equipped to ask
relevant questions regarding the chemotherapy. I
asked what stage I was in and what my CA-125

count was. The CA-125 is a blood test that tells you if you have ovarian cancer. Dr. Powell told me that my CA-125 count was 126 but needed to go down to below 30. He also said that I was in stage 1C. He gave me a good prognosis and said that I had a 90% chance of a full recovery. My mom and I prayed and thanked God for the good news! Dr. Powell recommended the chemo to ensure that any hidden cancer cells would be destroyed. He said that he would schedule me for six hours of chemo once a month for six months beginning November 5th. While I was relieved and grateful for the good prognosis, I was also dreading the chemo!

My mother was caring for me at home while I recovered from the surgery, but she would leave to run short errands during the day. The next day after having my staples removed, I was standing in the kitchen when I felt water running down my leg. This was quite alarming! I rushed to the bathroom where I continued to release water. It felt as though I had no control over my bladder and the water was pink which made me think it contained blood. I was home alone, and I began to panic. I called the doctor's office but had to leave a message and wait for someone to return my call. I tried calling my mother on her cell phone, but it went straight to voicemail. I remembered that my brother (who lives right down the street) was home until noon that day, so I called him.

I didn't know what was happening and I was scared to be alone. My brother came right over and stayed with me until my mother got home. The nurse returned my call and explained that it was most likely that some of my internal stitches had dissolved which had been holding back some fluid. She also said that I could have a bladder infection which a urine test later confirmed. She asked the doctor to prescribe an antibiotic. After one day everything cleared up.

Having a hysterectomy is major surgery and it takes a long time to fully recover. Not to mention that I was malnourished and dehydrated due to not eating anything except bites of crackers for six weeks prior to the surgery. I was very weak and even had difficulty walking. I did not have an appetite, and nothing sounded appealing. Dr. Powell warned me that I needed protein to build up my white blood cell count, but I could not bring myself to eat meat.

It took a couple of months, but I slowly regained my appetite. My education has taught me that sometimes you have to start by retraining your brain, so I started watching the Food Network and my mother made me homemade soups and stews. I began by just eating the broth and then the gravy and worked my way up to eating vegetables. Finally, after a couple of months I was able to eat meat.

I don't know why I had to go through this experience, but I know that it has made me more sympathetic to people who are ill. At one point, I felt so sick and the pain was so bad that I actually understood how people with terminal illnesses would think about ending the pain. I want to use my experience to help others make it through their own journeys.

On November 5, 2007, I started my first chemo treatment at the Zimmer Center. It was an all-day process and I spent six hours in the chemo chair hooked up to an IV. While I write about certain things that happened to me in this book, it is not to say that those things will happen to you. Everyone is different. All in all, the chemo was not as bad as I had anticipated, and the chemo nurses took excellent care of me. I was never left alone, and they took a personal interest in my comfort every time that I received a treatment. The following chapters are filled with information based on my experience and what I learned during my fight for survival...

TIP ONE: TREATMENT PLAN & POSSIBLE SIDE EFFECTS

When your cancer is first diagnosed, your doctor will review a treatment plan with you. This may involve surgery, radiation therapy, chemotherapy, hormone therapy, and biologic immunotherapy or some combination of those treatments. All of these regimes kill cells. In the process of killing the cancer cells, some healthy cells are also destroyed. That is what causes the side effects of the cancer treatments. You may experience any or none of the following:

- Sore mouth or throat or dry mouth

- Sores or white patches on your lips, mouth or throat
- Loss of appetite
- A change in sense of taste or smell
- Weight loss or weight gain
- Lactose intolerance
- Diarrhea
- Vomiting and nausea
- Stomach pain
- Constipation
- Pain or burning when you urinate
- Frequent urination
- Not being able to urinate
- Reddish or bloody urine
- Dental problems
- Fatigue
- Depression
- Acing in the bones
- Muscle, bone, or joint pain
- Weak, sore or achy muscles
- Rectal bleeding
- Shaking or trembling

- Hearing loss
- Itching or hives
- Severe skin rash
- Darkened, yellow, brittle or cracked nails
- Warmth or redness in your face, neck, arms or upper chest
- Swelling in your face or hands
- Swelling or tingling in your mouth or throat
- Tingling/numbing/burning sensation in your hands, arms, legs or feet
- Chest tightness
- Fast, slow, or uneven heartbeat
- Light-headedness or fainting
- Trouble breathing
- Bloody or black, tarry stools
- Changes in vision
- Fever, chills, or cough
- Ringing in your ears or trouble hearing
- Unusual bleeding, bruising or weakness
- Hair loss
- Anemia
- Confusion or memory loss

- Loss of balance or clumsiness
- Walking problems
- Jaw pain
- Onset of menopause/hormonal changes which may include hot flashes
- Infertility
- Earaches
- Headaches
- Impotence (for men)

Please note that some people don't experience any side effects. Everyone is different and many things factor into whether or not you will have side effects. These factors include the type of cancer you have, the part of your body being treated, the type and length of treatment, the dose of treatment, your diet, your personal outlook or attitude, and the medications you are taking to prevent side effects.

There are lots of medications being prescribed that can prevent almost any side effect out there. I experienced loss of appetite, weight loss, some lactose intolerance, some constipation, some fatigue (although not as bad as most), one bout of rectal bleeding due to eating popcorn, a one-time experience of numbness and tingling in my hands, arms, legs and feet, a one-time experience of feeling nauseous, hair loss, and aching in my bones. The worst of the side effects for me was the aching. This may have been due partly to the chemo, but it is mostly attributed to a side effect of a shot (Neulasta®), that I had to take after each chemo treatment to increase my white blood cell count. This shot caused terrible aching in my back, legs and feet. The aching usually lasted around four days. Generally, side effects disappear after your treatments stop.

TIP TWO: CA-125

When working on a project, I like to keep a record of progress. I created an excel spreadsheet so that I could monitor my blood cell count as well as the score for the ovarian cancer test. The CA-125 is a blood test which is an indicator for cancer. The blood contains substances at certain levels that are called tumor markers. When the tumor markers rise above a specified range, it may indicate cancer. Please note that tumor markers are not an absolute when predicting cancer, but they are a great tool for doctors to use.

The tests usually used for breast cancer are the CA 15-3 or the CA 27-29. The test for ovarian cancer is generally the CA-125. There is also another blood test called OvaSure® which was developed by Yale University researchers that claims to detect early-stage ovarian cancer with 99% accuracy.

My first CA-125 score was 126. It is supposed to be below 30 (between 4.0 – 30.2). After the surgery it came down to 32.1. After my first chemo treatment my score was 9.4 and after my last chemo treatment my score was 4. The chemo nurses told me that they could not believe how low my score was. They said there are people who have never had cancer that have scores higher than mine. I had a lot of people praying for me and I also followed my doctor's orders.

Along with recording the various scores from my CBC, I also kept track of my blood count related to when I took antibiotics. I took antibiotics five separate times while I was sick and while taking chemo. I noticed that each time that I took antibiotics, my white blood count was lower than the times that I was not taking them.

TIP THREE: SIDE EFFECTS OF CHEMO

My first chemo treatment was the hardest one for me. Three days after my fist treatment, I was standing in the kitchen when I began to feel sick. I felt nauseated and also like I was going to have diarrhea. At the same time, my whole body started to severely tingle almost like I was being zapped by a stun gun. I broke out into a cold sweat and my ears went shut which caused dizziness. It was a terrible feeling! However, my doctor had prescribed a pill (Prochlorperazine®) that was for nausea, so I took it immediately. I was already taking other medications prescribed for nausea, but this pill turned off nausea responses in the brain while the other nausea medication worked in the stomach.

I felt terrible for about half an hour and then the pill must have kicked in because I started feeling better. I kept track on a calendar of when I felt bad so that I could see if there was a pattern. That way I could be prepared and possibly block the nausea before it started. I took the Prochlorperazine® on the third day after each chemo treatment prior to feeling sick and it worked! As Barney Fife would say, "Nip it, nip it, nip it!"

Chemotherapy can also cause anemia. Anemia is the result of the bone marrow's inability to produce red blood cells. Red blood cells carry oxygen to every area of your body. If there are not enough red blood cells, then your body will not get enough oxygen to operate efficiently. Anemia can cause several symptoms and problems in and of itself. You may feel fatigued, feel like your heart is pounding and beating too fast, have shortness of breath, or feel dizzy or faint. There is a shot to stimulate your bone marrow to increase the

production of red blood cells just as there is a shot
to increase white blood cells. My problem was
insufficient white cells. Along with getting the
shot, you should have well-balanced meals, get
plenty of sleep, and don't attempt to do everything
yourself. Rest and accept help from friends and
family.

Along with the bone marrow's inability to
produce white and red blood cells, chemo can also
cause the bone marrow to stop or slow down the
production of platelets. Platelets are the blood cells
that help stop any bleeding by making blood clots.
If you do not have enough platelets, you will bleed
and bruise more easily. If your bone marrow is not
producing enough platelets, you may have
symptoms such as pinpoint red dots under your
skin, bruising, nose bleeds, gums bleeding, vaginal
bleeding, headaches, dark or bloody stool, pinkish
colored urine, and blurred or changes in your vision.
Blood work is always taken prior to administering
chemotherapy and a complete blood count is
included in that blood work. If your platelets are

too low, your doctor may offer medicine to stimulate your bone marrow to produce more platelets or he may suggest a platelet transfusion.

TIP FOUR: DO NOT EAT POPCORN!

I gave this tip a page all to itself because of its importance. I had a bad experience which has been attributed to eating popcorn the day before getting one of my chemo treatments. I thought that eating popcorn would be a good source of roughage which would help with digestion. Boy, was I wrong! The popcorn seemed to gather in my intestines where it hardened. A few days later after being constipated, I finally went to the bathroom but because the popcorn had hardened into big clusters in my intestines, it was very painful! About an hour later I started bleeding from the rectum. That was extremely upsetting and scary.

Everything always seemed to happen to me on the weekends when I could not reach my doctor. I did not know why I was bleeding. The bleeding started on a Friday night and continued until Monday afternoon. I was bleeding what appeared to be approximately a teaspoon of blood every half hour and I felt an urge to go to the bathroom every time I would bleed. That feeling alone was terrible.

I had been given a magnet with a 24-hour nurse line called Vitaline. At the time, I did not remember that this line also had a physician on-call 24-7. I called on a Saturday morning to see what I should do. The nurse that I spoke with advised me to go to the ER. Before taking her advice, I had the presence of mind to ask her two important questions. 1. Was I losing a dangerous amount of blood? And 2. What would they do to me if I went to the ER? She told me I was not in any danger with that amount of blood loss and I could wait until Monday to contact my doctor unless the bleeding got worse. She also let me know that if I went to the ER, I would be examined and scoped. I did not like the sound of that, so I decided to wait until Monday.

In the meantime, the nurse suggested that the bleeding might be caused by hemorrhoids. I never had hemorrhoids before, but she told me that they could be caused by the chemo weakening the walls of my intestines. She suggested that I try Tucks which might have helped if the bleeding wasn't internal. It turned out that I made the right decision because the bleeding stopped by Monday afternoon. I found out later, after talking to my doctor, that popcorn can have that affect if eaten shortly before or after taking chemo. It was several months before I ate popcorn again!

TIP FIVE: FOOD

When I went in for my first chemo treatment, I was bombarded with information given to me by the nurses. One benefit that Zimmer Center offered was the consultation services of a dietician. A good dietician can provide you with important information about what type of diet is best for you and may be able to answer questions for you throughout the duration of your chemo treatments. A balanced diet can also help with side effects such as fatigue. It was suggested to me that I limit my caffeine intake and increase protein.

Chemo lowers your immune system and makes you more susceptible to foodborne illnesses.

There is a greater risk of contracting E-Coli when consuming fresh fruits and vegetables. I was tempted to eat salads, but I resisted the temptation because I did not want to take the chance of getting sick. You can substitute things for fresh fruit like eating applesauce instead of apples or canned pineapple, peaches, etc. You can eat fresh vegetables as long as you cook them. I love steamed broccoli and cauliflower and they even have cancer-fighting agents in them. Additionally, when thawing meat, you should place it in the refrigerator and not the kitchen counter. It is important to cook meat and eggs thoroughly and avoid raw shellfish. Also, you should only consume pasteurized or processed juices and ciders as well as only pasteurized milk and cheese.

For the same reason to not eat fresh fruits and vegetables, you should also not eat fast foods or at buffets when undergoing chemo. It is a good idea to stay away from fast food restaurants anyway. This should be a time when you start eating healthier if you have not been eating that way previously.

My doctor and a nutritionist at the Zimmer Center recommended higher calorie foods with lots of protein. Dairy products such as milk and cheese are great unless you are lactose intolerant. Forget the diet foods and sugar-free foods. This is the time to build up your body so you can withstand the effects of the cancer and of the treatments. You may not feel like eating a lot, so make a point to eat foods that are higher in calories. Some higher calorie food suggestions include: pancakes, cinnamon buns, doughnuts, cheeseburgers (but not from fast-food restaurants), grilled cheese sandwiches, milk-based soups, potato salad, biscuits, most meat, ice cream, milkshakes, cake, pie, and cookies.

While I am on the subject of food, I will include something that I learned from experience regarding what to eat around the time of each chemo treatment. I found that I felt much better if I only ate soft food or liquids like soup a few days prior to and a few days after each chemo treatment.

The chemo made everything I ate harden up during digestion. I would have a couple of days of constipation and that uncomfortable feeling that accompanies it around each chemo treatment. Although it was uncomfortable, I did not experience any rectal bleeding except for the popcorn incident. I just felt a lot better when I only ate soup or pudding or other soft foods during those few days. It took me a while to learn this, so I hope this tip will help you.

This leads right into the topic of using a stool softener. I recommend Senokot because it did not cause bloating or gas and it is a natural vegetable laxative. I did not need it every month but definitely used it after eating the popcorn! I suggest taking 2 pills once a day for however many days you feel you need it but be sure to follow the directions on the bottle. One of the chemo nurses said that some people take as many as four a day.

Chemo treatments can cause constipation in some people and some medications can also cause constipation. It is important to drink plenty of fluids to keep your stool soft. The usual recommendation is at least eight 8-ounce glasses per day. Increasing the fiber in your diet can also help but be sure to check with your doctor first because a high fiber diet is not recommended for certain types of cancer. Exercise can also help to keep you regulated.

Mouth sores, tender gums, and a sore throat or esophagus often result from radiation or chemotherapy. If this happens, you should consult with your doctor because it could be due to an unrelated dental problem and your doctor may be able to give you medicine that will help to control mouth and throat pain. Be aware that certain foods may irritate an already tender mouth or make chewing difficult.

As I stated earlier, I went on a soft food or liquid diet a few days prior to my chemo treatment and continued it for a few days after. I did not have any trouble with mouth or throat sores, but the soft diet helped with digestion. On the same note, you will want to avoid citrus fruits such as oranges, grapefruit, lemons, and spicy or salty foods.

Some foods you may want to include are:

- Instant mashed potatoes
- Milkshakes
- Applesauce or canned peaches
- Cottage cheese or yogurt
- Macaroni and cheese
- Custards, puddings and gelatin
- Ice cream
- Scrambled eggs
- Oatmeal

Additionally, you should stay away from sugar-free foods. Sorbitol, which is a sugar substitute that is used in many sugar-free foods, can cause diarrhea. I made the mistake of eating some sugar-free ice cream which caused cramping and diarrhea. Sugar-free gum can do the same thing. This isn't the time to be dieting so ditch the sugar-free foods.

Finally, it is important to drink a lot of water. Water keeps the body lubricated but it also plumps up your veins. When you receive chemo, it makes your veins shrink and hide making it difficult for the nurses to find a vein to draw blood or administer the chemo. Water helps fatten up the veins so drink a lot of water prior to any blood tests or chemo treatments. Drinking eight 8-ounce glasses of water a day is a good thing anyway. This is just another reason to drink a lot of water.

TIP SIX: LOSS OF APPETITE

Most people lose their appetite at some point during the duration of their chemo treatments. However, some people actually may gain weight. While most women do not like to think about gaining weight, it can be a good thing when you are taking chemo. You may lose your appetite due to the chemo treatments or even due to anxiety. Everyone reacts differently. I am a Licensed Professional Counselor and have seen people lose their appetite due to fear, anxiety, and depression. All of these emotions are normal when you are battling cancer. You may also experience a change in taste or smell which can influence your appetite.

I was sick for six weeks prior to having surgery to remove a large ovarian tumor. During that time, I lost my appetite because I was experiencing stomach pain and diarrhea. After surgery, I still did not have an appetite and my stomach was very sensitive. I explained some of this in the introduction of the book, so I won't go into detail again. My doctor prescribed two medications for me. One was supposed to help in the digestion process (Acipehx® in pill form) and the other one was to increase my appetite (Megestrol Acetate® in liquid form). I have to confess that I only took one dose of Megestrol Acetate® because I hated the taste. The way that I regained my appetite was by watching the Food Network and giving myself time to heal.

Even my favorite foods like bread and chocolate did not appeal to me and the thought of eating meat was disgusting! I knew that I needed to eat meat because I needed the protein to build up my white blood cells. I started by eating homemade chicken and beef soups. I only ate the broth at first and then I ate some vegetables. Next, I ate some beef stew. Once again, I only ate the gravy and vegetables. I kept watching food programs and pretty soon food started looking good.

One thing that may help is to try some of the food that you used to enjoy when you were a kid. I used to like Chef Boyardee Beef Ravioli. It has processed meat which isn't the healthiest thing to eat but it got me started eating meat again. As I continued watching the Food Network, I slowly regained my appetite. This process is an example of Cognitive Behavior Therapy. First you change your thinking (cognitive) and then your behavior will follow. Some other ideas that may help you with your appetite include:

- Have foods on hand that appealed to you when you were a child
- Keep snacks on hand. I began with Cheez-Its
- Remember that you can get protein from other sources such as peanut butter
- Liquid meals are an option such as Ensure

- Sometimes cold food is more appealing like pudding, yogurt, or popsicles
- Exercise stimulates the appetite

TIP SEVEN: NAUSEA

There are many different medications that
can help with nausea. My doctor prescribed three
different medications. Dexamethasone® which is a
steroid that helps prevent nausea and Ondansetron®
which works on both the peripheral and central
nerves. It reduces the activity of the vagus nerve,
which activates the vomiting center in the medulla
oblongata (the lower portion of the brain stem) and
serotonin receptors. These were given to me in an
IV prior to each chemo treatment and in a pill form.
I was told to take five tablets of Dexamethasone®
at 10:00 the night before taking chemo and five
more tablets at 6:00 the morning of my chemo

treatment. I was also prescribed to take one tablet of Ondansetron® at bedtime on the night of my chemo treatment and continue taking it twice a day for three days after my chemo treatment.

In addition, Prochlorperazine® was prescribed to be used as needed when I felt nauseated after chemo treatments. It acts by blocking dopamine receptors. Basically, the brain has neurotransmitters that send messages to your stomach which can cause the nauseated feeling. Prochlorperazine® blocked those messages and really worked for me.

I only felt nauseated once a few days after my first chemo treatment. It was a horrible feeling because it was combined with other side effects such as breaking out in a cold sweat, feeling dizzy, having severe tingling which felt like an electric shock in my whole body, and a lot of pressure in my ears. At the first sign of feeling sick, I took Prochlorperazine® and about half an hour later, I felt better. However, if your medications are not working for you, tell your doctor and try the same things you would do it you had the stomach flu. Try eating crackers, toast, ice chips, carbonated drinks like ginger ale, yogurt, or rice. Sometimes sucking on a mint candy can help. Other techniques you may want to try, include breathing deeply and slowly when you feel nauseated and using relaxation therapy.

TIP EIGHT: HYGIENE

It will make you feel better if you take a lot of showers. This may sound like common sense, but I have included this tip because when you are taking chemo you lose your energy and it is easy to stay in your pajamas all day. Sometimes you have to push yourself to get moving or even to take a shower. But after you take a shower or a bath you always feel better. There is something refreshing about feeling clean and smelling good. It is also nice to feel the sensation of the warm water. In addition, taking a hot bath or shower can help you relax and sleep better.

Part of good hygiene is washing your hands,

but it is especially important to remember to wash your hands when you are taking chemo treatments because your immune system is compromised during that time and you are more susceptible to germs and illness. I was told that I should not clean or even be around any litter boxes, bird cages, or fish tanks. I was also told not to have close contact with other people such as shaking hands or hugging people in church. Most germs are passed by touching someone or something. That is why it is so important to wash your hands a lot.

Washing your hands all the time tends to make them dry. Buy a good moisturizer for your hands to keep the skin from cracking making you more vulnerable to germs. Buy an extra tube to keep in your purse or the car.

Chemo generally dries out the mucus membrane in your body such as the inside of your nose and mouth. I put Vaseline in my nostrils at night to keep them from drying and bleeding. I am prone to nosebleeds, but never had one during the six months that I was taking chemo. As long as I knew the possibility of what to expect or what could happen, I took precautions to prevent it.

When you are undergoing chemo treatments, you have little resistance to fight off the germs like you normally would. During that time, I had a parrot and a cat. While I was receiving treatments, my mother took over my chores of cleaning the bird cage and the litter box. I was very fortunate to have such a wonderful mother. I was very careful to do my best to follow the hygiene rules, so I did not complicate the situation.

I did not even go out of the house very much during the six months that I was taking chemo. I would sit in my secluded backyard a lot and enjoy the natural setting. I did go out a few times around Christmas, but I stayed away from people as much as possible. I did not go anywhere where I would be in an enclosed place with people for any period of time. I didn't go to church or to the theater. I didn't get in cars with anyone other than my mother and I asked that friends and family not come over if they were not feeling well. I felt bad enough with

what I was going through without making it worse
by getting a cold or the flu which could have turned
into something much worse due to having a low
resistance. I was fortunate that I did not catch
anything during that time, but I also remembered to
keep washing my hands.

When you are manicuring your finger and
toenails, flossing your teeth, and shaving, be careful
not to cut yourself. Also, do not pinch or squeeze
pimples. Don't scratch yourself too hard or rub
yourself too roughly when you are drying off after a
shower. And if you do accidently get cut, clean the
wound right away with soap and antiseptic. Also,
don't get any immunizations while taking chemo.
And stay away from standing water which can
breed germs such as bird baths, humidifiers, and
public bathroom sinks.

It is also important to remember to take care
of your teeth when you are undergoing chemo
treatments. There were days when I did not feel
like doing anything including brushing my teeth.
However, I did not want more problems than I

already had, so I flossed and brushed regularly. The one thing I skipped while on chemo was rinsing with a mouthwash. Most mouthwashes contain alcohol which can really burn your mouth if it is dry from the chemo. You may want to use a soft toothbrush and rinse your mouth with warm water if your gums are sore. You can also use a mouthwash with sodium bicarbonate (baking soda) which should not irritate your gums.

TIP NINE: HAIR

Chemo often causes your hair to fall out. I had long blond hair and hated to cut it, so I just let it fall out, which happened after the third round of chemo. This was a mistake because my hair was everywhere. I had to pick it off of my clothes constantly and it filled the vacuum when I would sweep. I was not that upset about losing my hair because I knew it would grow back. My focus was on getting well. I had been very sick and barely able to eat for six weeks before my diagnosis. Because I had been sick for so long, I just wanted to feel better so looks were not as important.

However, there was one instance when I

looked in the mirror and began to cry. My hair was falling out in clumps. It was Thanksgiving and my family was gathering at my brother's house just down the street from where we lived. I was going to attend but when I looked in the mirror, I suddenly felt very depressed and decided not to attend. I think I might not have felt so bad if I had gotten my hair cut before it fell out. It would have given me a little control over the situation.

I have always had a sensitive scalp, but it became extremely tender when I was going through chemo. It seemed to be especially tender when I was losing my hair. It hurt to even lay my head on a pillow. If this happens to you, buy a mild shampoo or even a baby shampoo and wash your scalp with it when you shower. It made my scalp feel better.

Speaking of losing your hair and a tender scalp, a lot of heat escapes through your head so if you don't have hair, it can make you quite cold. I started losing my hair in November and even though I live in the south, the temperatures were starting to drop. My scalp was very tender when I was in the process of losing my hair so at that time, I preferred to wear stocking caps around the house. They kept my head warm and were soft on my scalp.

I decided to look into getting a wig and ended up buying a moderately priced wig at a local shop. It looked pretty good but since it was not actual hair, it made my head hot and itchy. You can buy special wigs with gel on the inside that are much cooler to wear. You cannot always find them in wig shops, but most wig catalogs carry them. I bought one from a Paula Young catalog that was made with "Coolmax Fabric" which they advertise to provide "soothing, itch-free wear and maximum breathability." If you invest in this type of wig you will most likely feel more comfortable.

Since I had just moved to a new town, nobody knew me except for my family so most of the time I just wore a lot of different baseball caps when I went out. As I mentioned earlier, I did not have a job, so I did not need to dress up. It is also good to know that some health insurance policies cover the cost of a wig if your hair loss is due to chemo treatments. In addition, your wig is a tax-deductible expense.

TIP TEN: WHITE BLOOD CELLS

Having cancer may lower your white blood cell count. This does not happen to everyone, but it did happen to me. When you receive chemo treatments, your white blood cell count has to be at a certain level, or it is too dangerous to get the treatment. Therefore, prior to each chemo treatment, they will test your blood to make sure you have enough white blood cells. If your white blood cells are not high enough, you will be given a shot to increase them. Additionally, the chemo decreases your white blood cells.

I had to get a shot (Neulasta®) each month a day after receiving the chemo treatment to increase my white blood cell count. This is not uncommon. I was also told that taking antibiotics may decrease your white blood cell count although, I'm not sure if this is a fact or not. However, I had taken several rounds of antibiotics during this ordeal and my white blood cell count was below the normal range even before I started my chemo treatments.

Neulasata® has a side-affect that some people experience. One to two days after receiving the shot, the bones in my legs, feet, and back would ache. The ache was extreme, and nothing seemed to help. I tried soaking my feet in hot water and rubbing them, but nothing helped. Then one day while receiving my chemo, I overheard a nurse say that Duke University was doing a study on Claritin® and they were finding that it helped to relieve some of the aching caused by Neulasta®. I tried it and it worked!

I started taking Claritin® the evening of the day that I received the Neulasta® shot and continued to take one a day for the next several days until the aching stopped. In my experience, the aching usually started one to two days after I received the shot and it lasted three to four days.

Claritin® did not totally eliminate the aching but it really helped a lot!

Another thing that helps with the aching is to try to stay off of your feet as much as possible during the timeframe mentioned above. I made the mistake of taking a long walk a day after getting the shot since exercise was recommended. However, this made the aching worse. I found that I felt the best if I just laid in bed and took Claritin® for a few days. This is not to say that you should stay in bed all of the time. Do what feels best for you but it may be best to plan your exercise around the time when any side effects from Neulasta® have passed.

As I mentioned previously, I had a low white blood cell count even before my first chemo treatment. It had never been a problem before, but it is possible that having cancer made it low. I researched the internet and asked my doctor what I could do to increase my white blood cell count and the only answer besides getting a shot was to eat protein. A normal white blood cell count range is from 4.6 to 10.2. My count started at 4.7 and went as low as 2.2.

TIP ELEVEN: DEPRESSION

Crying is a way to release your emotions and it can be a good thing to do as long as you do not wallow in your sorrows. I had times when I really felt sorry for myself. I felt helpless and I questioned God. I couldn't understand why this was happening to me. I allowed myself some time to be sad, but I reminded myself that there were others who had it much worse than I. I started thinking of ways that I might be able to help others who were going through what I was. I also started counting my blessings. Every time I thought of something negative, I replaced it with a positive. When I thought about all the medical bills that were piling up and how I did not have a job, I thought about how nice it was not to have to worry about trying to take care of myself while having to work.

When you are told that you have cancer, the world stops spinning for a moment. Time just stands still as you are hit in the face with something you just cannot grasp. Cancer is something that happens to other people, not to me! I have been healthy all of my life. This cannot be true! But when the doctor looks you in the eye and tells you that it *is* true, you are slapped in the face by reality.

After denial, came a feeling of hopelessness. Since I have cancer, my life must be over. At the time that I was diagnosed, the doctor did not know my prognosis until he opened me up. He was basing his diagnosis on a CT scan and on the results of a blood test.

In my case, the CT scan revealed that I had a basketball sized tumor which was elongated throughout my abdomen. Dr. Powell is a full professor at UNC-Chapel Hill and one of the nation's leading gynecological oncologists, so he knew (based on his experience and expertise) that it was ovarian cancer.

The night in the hospital before my surgery was very scary. I did not know what to expect. I didn't know if the cancer had spread throughout my body or even if I would survive the surgery. All of those thoughts kept swirling around in my head. My mother and brother stayed with me in my hospital room as long as they were allowed but after they left, I was alone with those thoughts. That was the worst night of my life. I admit that I cried a lot that night. I cried out of fear and sorrow for myself. We all have our moments of weakness. It is part of being human.

Chemo zaps the body of energy and when you are fatigued, depression often follows. If you have been given a less than perfect prognosis, undergoing months of chemotherapy or radiation, feeling sick, hate the way you look because of hair loss or bloating, it is easy to become depressed. The most important thing to do is not to give up hope. Believe in a positive outcome and believe in yourself. Decide that you are going to do everything possible to beat the cancer.

It is also important to talk about your feelings. This may be the most fearful and anxiety ridden time of your life. It is great to have a friend or family member to talk to, but it is even better to be able to talk to a nurse, a therapist or another cancer patient. That is one reason why it is helpful to join a cancer/chemo support group. Eating a good diet, exercising, and getting enough rest are also important for good mental health. Try to stay away from stressful situations as much as possible. Stress is one of the worst things to have in your life, especially now. Think of little things that make you happy and surround yourself with as many of them as you can. Sometimes just having flowers in your room can change your mood.

Read positive and uplifting books and watch a lot of comedies. Think of ways you can help someone else. Listen to your favorite music. Don't focus on the negatives. Keep believing in miracles and keep praying. God is listening! If you do not understand something about your treatment or recovery, write down your questions and ask your doctor at your next appointment. Empower yourself with knowledge.

I'm a true believer that laughter is the best medicine. My brother and sister-in-law bought me a portable DVD player with headphones which I took with me each time that I went for a chemo treatment. It was a good distraction while I sat there for six hours. I watched funny movies and some old-time sitcoms which I bought ahead of time. One movie that I highly recommend is *Evan Almighty* starring Steve Carrell. It is not only funny but has a great message (i.e., have faith).

The sitcoms I bought were helpful because they were old ones from when I was a kid and they brought back good memories as I watched them. I was probably the only one in the chemo room who was laughing while I was receiving chemo. It really is good to take your mind off of your troubles and just try to relax. My friends and family bought me funny movies that I could watch at home while I was recuperating. It gave us something to do together and kept us laughing instead of focusing on my condition.

TIP TWELVE: KEEP A
POSITIVE ATTITUDE

When we are sick it is easy to sink into depression. It is hard to be happy when you don't feel good. When you are given a cancer diagnosis and know that the road ahead will be a difficult one, it is easy to focus on the pain and anxiety of what lies ahead. Remember to take one step at a time. In the comedy movie, *"What About Bob?"* the psychiatrist wrote a book called 'Baby Steps.' It is a very funny movie, but it is also very true. Don't jump to conclusions and picture negative outcomes.

I had heard all kinds of horror stories about chemo which filled me with dread. You have to take one day at a time or "baby steps." I had many scary and upsetting things happen, but all in all, the chemo was not as bad as I had anticipated. Try to think positive thoughts and plan little things that make you happy. Plan to do something fun after your chemo treatments are finished so you have something to look forward to. Remember that there is new research going on all of the time and a new treatment for you may be just around the corner. Doctors and researchers have made so many advances over the past 40 years. My grandmother had colon cancer 40 years ago and she really suffered with her chemo treatments. Things are so much better today. Keep praying and believing in miracles. They still happen.

However, for those of you who have difficulty believing in miracles, let me give you something else to consider. When you are given a diagnosis of cancer, your emotions generally take over. You feel fragile because you are vulnerable. That fear may play a significant role in your susceptibility to disease and even to your recovery. But all is not lost. You have a choice in how you feel. You control the way you think and in turn control your emotions which can help or hinder your recovery.

The central nervous system and the immune system communicate with each other. Immune cells travel in your blood through your body and come in contact with all the other cells. If the immune cells recognize other cells, they leave them alone. But if they do not recognize certain cells, they attack them. Therefore, if the immune cell comes into contact with a cancer cell, it will attack it unless it misidentifies it. The field that studies the correlation between the immune system and the central nervous system is called psychoneuroimmunology.

Research has found that the chemical messengers that function broadly in the brain and immune system are the chemical messengers that are most dense in the neural regions that control emotion. They have actually identified a contact point where nerve cells release neurotransmitters which regulate immune cells. What all of this means is that your emotions directly relate to your immune system. Therefore, when you are extremely anxious or depressed, it can compromise your immune function to the point that it can speed the metastasis of cancer. That information should open your eyes to the reality that your mental attitude plays a part in your recovery.

TIP THIRTEEN: SUPPORT GROUPS

Some of your best support may come from being involved in a cancer support group. You will meet other men and women who are going through some of the same things that you are going through. They will have a lot of important information they can share with you and maybe you will be able to help one of them. Someone in that group may be able to answer some of your questions that even the doctors or nurses may not be able to answer due to firsthand experience. They might think to tell you something helpful that the doctors might have forgotten to mention such as "don't eat popcorn!" It is also good for your spirit to talk to people who are going through the same thing you are, so you do not feel so alone. And you may make a friend who

will be there for you on a weekend when you may
not be able to reach your doctor with a question.

I tend to want to be alone when I don't feel
well. I want to stay in bed and isolate myself until I
feel better. That may be okay when you have flu
but when you have cancer, it is better to connect
with a support group over the duration. Knowledge
is power and support groups provide firsthand
knowledge. Also, you can join a group just by
talking on the phone if you don't feel like attending
a meeting or distance is an issue. In addition,
studies have shown that social isolation doubles the
chances of sickness.

TIP FOURTEEN: 24-HOUR EMERGENCY HOTLINE

It was my luck that when something bad happened, it always happened on the weekend when I couldn't reach my doctor. If you are like me, it is scary when something strange happens to your body. When I was going through this time, I was inclined to become alarmed and worry that the situation was worse than it was. One time my port became infected and I had a fever of 102. This started on a Friday night. Another time I had rectal bleeding which also started on a Friday night. Those were just two examples.

Fortunately, New Hampshire Medical Center had provided me with a 24-hour nurse hotline called Vitaline which also provides contact with an on-call physician 24-7. Always be prepared for things to happen on the weekend. If you are starting to feel bad or starting to have a problem on a Thursday or Friday, don't put off making a phone call to your doctor. Things always seem to get worse on the weekend when you may not be able to reach your doctor. Just call to see if you need to do something before your situation worsens. And remember to ask if there is a 24-hour hotline that you can use.

TIP FIFTEEN: GETTING A PORT

Getting a port is a good option for a lot of people. However, for me, it was not a pleasant experience. A port is also known as a vascular access device. If you receive chemo intravenously, it makes your veins shrink and hide. This makes it difficult for the nurses to find a vein when they need to insert an IV.

I had been sick for six weeks prior to my diagnosis and during that time, my stomach felt like it was burning whenever I drank a sip of water. Therefore, I did not drink much water for six weeks. Because of that, I was severely dehydrated and finding my veins was next to impossible. I was not informed about ports before I started the chemo treatments. I had envisioned sitting in a chair with an IV inserted in my arm. That is not usually how it is done.

If you only need a couple of chemo treatments, they may not suggest a port, but most people need more than two treatments so in many cases a port is used. If you are given an IV without the use of a port, the nurse will try to find a vein near your wrist or in your hand. The nurses do not use the crook of your arm because they do not want the needle breaking off or coming out if you bend your arm.

My doctor ordered six chemo treatments of Paclitaxel® and Carboplatin® (one treatment a month for six months). My treatments were an all-day affair. I would go in around 8:30 in the morning and have blood drawn and have an IV inserted (for the times that I did not have the port). Then I would see my doctor for a quick exam and answer a few questions regarding how I was feeling and if I was having any side effects from the chemo. Also, during that time, I was attended to by one of Dr. Powell's nurses. All of his nurses are kind and empathetic. One nurse in particular (Melinda) was always upbeat and helpful. She continually let me know how much she cared by her kind words and encouragement.

After my exam with the doctor, I would go to the chemo room where I would wait until the results of my blood work came back from the lab. Once they had the results, they would hook me up to the IV and I would sit for approximately six hours before it was finished. The nurses had a very difficult time finding my veins. The first time I went in for chemo, the nurse searched my lower arms, wrists and back of my hands and stuck me several times before she hit the mark. This nurse was very kind and compassionate and did her best to make me comfortable, but my hands are very sensitive.

My first chemo treatment was given by IV inserted in a vein in my right hand. The chemo nurses were very kind and helpful. They suggested that I get a port because it would be a one-time procedure to insert the port which would eliminate the need to find a vein every time that I came in to get a treatment.

I must admit that the thought of having a port inserted under my skin really disgusted me. I had seen a lady with a port protruding out of her chest (near her neck) and it looked awful. It looked like something from a sci fi movie. However, everyone assured me that it was no big deal and I would be much happier after I had the port. I reluctantly agreed but something about it made me very anxious.

Getting a port did not seem like a simple procedure to me. The whole thing takes several hours. You have a choice of having it placed under your skin in your chest or your arm. The port is a catheter which is surgically inserted into a tube that is pulled from a vein in your arm or chest through to a larger vein in your chest which leads to your heart. The larger the vein that is used, the less chance that it will be destroyed by the chemo. Also, the larger veins carry the blood faster. The port is approximately the size of a half dollar. The middle of the port is rubbery and can be punctured with a needle that is specially designed to connect with the IV tubing. The port can then be used for blood tests, IVs and even medications so you don't have to be continually stuck with needles.

You are prepped for the surgical procedure and an IV is inserted for the anesthesia. Some of my anxiety was due to the fact that my veins were hiding and once again it was difficult for the nurse to find a vein to insert the IV. I admit that I am a big baby when it comes to needles so keep in mind that you will probably have a much better experience if you keep a positive attitude.

The anesthesia puts you into a twilight feeling and you are not completely put out, but you don't feel any pain. A local anesthetic is used. The procedure is usually performed in radiology where they can use a type of x-ray machine to see what they are doing when they insert and thread the tube. The actual procedure takes about half an hour. I remember the radiologist talking to me while he did the procedure, but I kept my eyes shut because I didn't want to see what was happening.

My problem began shortly after the procedure. When they had finished the procedure, the nurse applied a type of glue that helps hold the skin together. The problem was that the nurse did not wait for the glue to dry before he put the bandages on. The bandage adhered to my skin so after several days when I was supposed to take off the bandage, part of it would not come off. I called the radiologist and asked what I should do about the bandage and I was told to leave it on and eventually it would fall off. That is what I did, however, I think this is when the area became infected.

The bandage eventually fell off, but a day later the area on my arm around the port became red and began to hurt. Once again, this happened on a weekend when it would have been difficult to reach my doctor. I developed a fever and I was warned not to mess around if the wound became infected since the port led to my heart. I was also under the impression that they may not be able to give me the rest of the chemo treatments if I did not use a port. So, I was very upset and concerned when it became infected.

It was a Saturday, so I went to the local ER. The doctor in the ER had never worked with ports so he did not know what to do. This was at my local hospital (not at New Hanover). The ER doctor ended up calling another doctor who said I should be put on antibiotics. However, he scared me because he said I might have to have the port removed due to the infection. This news was upsetting because at that time I thought that there weren't any options for getting the chemo and I would not be able to receive the rest of my treatments. But that was not the case. When you first get the port, they put you on antibiotics for a week while you heal. Three days after I finished taking the first round of antibiotics, my port became infected. Four days after taking the second round of antibiotics, I started feeling better and my arm started to look better. But there was a small area in my arm that would not heal.

There was a small hole in my arm where the port was inserted that just would not close. Two weeks after receiving the port, I went back to the radiologist so he could look at my arm to see why it was not healing. He said it looked pretty good and to just give it more time to heal.

When I first got the port, I was told to not get the area wet and not to let the area rub against anything. The port was inserted on the inside of my upper left arm. That meant that I had to hold my arm out away from my body all of the time. I was supposed to let the air get to it so I did not have it bandaged. I had to sleep in one position with my arm on a pillow and try not to move it all night long. I had to take sponge baths instead of showers, so I did not get it wet. And it was winter, and I could not wear a sleeve on that arm. This went on for two and a half months!

My back ached from having to hold my arm out away from my body and I was cold all of the time because I could not wear anything on that arm. I got to use the port twice before it became infected again and I had to have it removed. After they removed the port, I had to return to the hospital four times to have the area cleaned and bandaged due to the infection.

I was able to receive my last three chemo treatments in a vein in my hand. I went through all of that pain and aggravation for two and a half months only to be able to use the port twice! Some people opt to get another port inserted if the first one becomes infected. I was given that option but did not want to take the chance that the second port might become infected.

Maybe if I had complained more to my doctor, things might have been different, but I did not want to be a complainer and did not think that there might be another option. Sometimes we need to be our own advocate and speak up. Doctors cannot read our minds and may not realize what we are experiencing unless we tell them.

TIP SIXTEEN: ANTIBIOTICS

Some antibiotics can cause allergic reactions and if severe, can cause a fever. When my port became infected for the second time, my local doctor prescribed Septra DS® which is a strong antibiotic. It turns out that I am allergic to it but at the time I did not know it. I had been taking it for eight days when I woke up one morning covered in a red rash and my face was bright red. I was aching and I had a fever of 102. I called a nurse at the Zimmer Center and she said that I needed to come in right away. Before I went in, I called my local doctor who suggested that I might be having an allergic reaction to the antibiotic. He told me to stop taking it which I did. I still went to the Zimmer Center to see the nurse and she ordered some blood work. She said she did not believe it was an allergic reaction since I had a fever. As it turned out, it was a severe allergic reaction to the antibiotic. In some cases, a severe allergic reaction can cause a fever. A day after I quit taking it, I was fine.

TIP SEVENTEEN: ACCEPT HELP

I always hate asking for help. I try to be self-sufficient. However, sometimes you need to ask for help. I was fortunate to have my mother who nursed me back to health. However, she was 80 years old at that time and she needed support too. My mother and I had just moved to North Carolina, so we did not have a big support group. Fortunately, we moved to be near my brother and his family, and he provided a lot of help. My brother (the Rev. Dr. William G. Waun) took me to my first couple of chemo treatments which were an hour and a half away. He did this until I was well enough to drive myself. He also came to my rescue on more than one occasion. My sister-in-law (Cynthia) researched my condition on the internet and provided me with information and questions that I could ask my doctor. My friends sent flowers, cards, and letters.

My mother did the most for me. She went to every chemo treatment with me. She made me homemade soups and stews when I didn't want to eat. She ran to the grocery store and bought me whatever I needed or wanted. She sat with me, laughed with me, cried with me, and prayed with me. I don't know what I would have done without her. Accept the help and love that others offer. You can pay it back or pay it forward when you feel better.

TIP EIGHTEEN:
FINANCIAL ASSISTANCE

I had an unusual situation because my job had ended along with my insurance coverage when I moved to North Carolina. I have never gone without health insurance even though I have been very healthy all of my life. I was paying for my own health insurance and thank God that I hadn't let it lapse! However, the one thing that I did change was that I decided to make my annual deduction higher and also selected a plan where the percentage I paid was higher so my monthly payments would be lower.

I had only been in North Carolina for a few days when I started to get sick. When I first became ill, I was covered under the policy that I had purchased in another state prior to moving for the first month. Then it switched to my North Carolina policy. The problem was that I had to meet the other state deductible in November and then meet the North Carolina deductible in December. Then I had to pay another North Carolina deductible in January because it was a new year! Besides all of the deductibles, I had to pay 30% of my medical expenses. Thirty percent may not sound like that much but when you are dealing with hospital stays and shots that cost $7,000 each, it really adds up! On top of that, I was unemployed, so I did not have an income.

One day while I was sitting in the chemo chair, I heard one of the chemo nurses telling another patient about how to get financial help. When she came over to check on me, I asked her about it, and she told me about a program that the hospital has. She even went and got me the paperwork to apply. After I applied, I waited for a few weeks but was fortunate to receive a letter stating that I had been approved through March. That was wonderful news since March 24th was my final chemo treatment.

This particular financial assistance program did not pay for everything associated with the hospital. I still had to pay for each doctor visit and for anything associated with radiology such as getting the port. But my insurance paid for 70% of those things so at least I was not responsible for as much. It was a huge relief to receive this financial help form the hospital since I was not eligible for any government help. So, if you are in need of financial help, it can't hurt to ask if your hospital has a financial assistance program.

CORRESPONDING THERAPIES

There are many other types of therapy you can receive while taking chemotherapy which can help you through this difficult time. They can help with the healing of your mind and body while reducing stress and easing side-effects. As a licensed professional counselor, I highly recommend counseling therapy. Counseling can include many other therapies such as journaling, art therapy, imagery, rhythmic breathing, and visualization. I also suggest the following:

Massage Therapy: The Zimmer Center where I received my chemo treatments offered massage therapy during my treatment. Massage therapy uses different styles of touch, stroking and manipulation of the muscles to help you relax and release tension.

100

Pet Therapy: The Zimmer Center also offered pet therapy. During chemo treatments a pet therapist would come for a visit with a dog. This is an animal that has been trained to work with sick or injured people. The pet therapist would walk the dog around the chemo room and ask patients if they would like to pet or talk to the dog. Animals are generally accepting of anyone. They do not judge us by our looks or loss of hair. It is comforting to touch a dog or cat and have them relate to you. It has even been proven that stroking a cat or dog can decrease your blood pressure.

Biofeedback: Biofeedback teaches you how to control different body functions such as blood pressure, heart rate, breathing, and muscle tension that used to be considered involuntary. This is usually done with the use of a machine where you can learn by watching monitoring instruments attached to your body that record changes in your physiology. Then, eventually, you will have a better self-regulation without the aid of those devices. There are also other means of reading biofeedback such as a chemically coated card which detects rises and falls in your skin temperature or hormonal changes. Biofeedback is a good tool to help you when you are tense and anxious and need to learn how to relax.

Progressive relaxation: This is a method where you sit in a comfortable chair or lay down in a quiet atmosphere. You slowly take a deep breath and concentrate on the muscles in your feet. Contract and relax those muscles and then exhale. You continue to breath while contracting and relaxing muscles in your legs and on up in your body finishing with the muscles in your face. Each time that you exhale and release your muscles, you release tension and relax that part of your body.

Visualization: I mentioned visualization earlier but want to touch on it again because many people use it to fight cancerous tumors. By using visualization, you can picture the tumor in your mind and think of the chemotherapy as soldiers or bombs crashing into the tumor to destroy it. You can create whatever picture you want to use and imagine it often throughout the day as you think about eliminating the cancer.

Reframing and Thought Stopping:

Reframing is changing the way you talk to yourself. It is a conscious change of an automatic thought from something negative or unrealistic to something positive, neutral, or objective. Thought stopping is interrupting your thoughts by ordering them to stop. When you feel anxious or upset, this is a sign that your thoughts are making you feel that way. If you have a belief about something such as, "I know I will get sick whenever I have a chemo treatment," this is jumping to a conclusion. You may not get sick every time that you have a chemo treatment and in fact, you may not get sick at all. But when you have those kinds of thoughts, they add to your anxiety and stress. The way to change those thoughts and consequential feelings is to use thought stopping. You can combine your thought stopping with reframing to improve the way that you feel. In other words, when you are anxious or worried about something, your body will usually cue you by making your heart beat faster or you will get sweaty palms. When you have these types of cues, think about what is going on in your head. If you are having negative or unrealistic thoughts or jumping to conclusions, then tell yourself to stop. Realize what you are doing to yourself. Then use reframing to replace that negative thought with one this is more realistic or objective.

Hypnosis: The use of hypnosis can help to reduce pain and anxiety. Hypnosis places you in a deep relaxed state of mind. A qualified hypnotist may be able to help you with many side effects.

Prayer and Meditation: For me, having ongoing communication with God is something I do throughout the day every day. The first thing that I did when I received my diagnosis was to pray. I know God is in control of my life and I cried out to Him for His help. Every time I was scared or uncertain, I prayed. When I felt alone, I prayed. I continue to pray and listen for His answers. I am fortunate in that I have many Christian friends and family members who prayed with me and for me during my crisis. My brother who is a priest anointed me with oil and prayed for my healing. Don't underestimate the power of prayer. Along with prayer there is meditation. Meditation is a form of relaxing and being quiet or listening. By being quiet and focusing on something specific such as killing the cancer cells or listening for an answer from God, you are freeing your mind from distractions and releasing stress from your body.

My prayer for you is that you will use this time in your life to stop any negative behavior and replace it with a renewed spirit. I hope that you will read this book and use it as you go through your own journey and that it will help you along the way. I believe that God wanted me to stop and pay attention to Him. I usually have to learn things the hard way in life, but once I learn a lesson, I remember it! God has opened my eyes to the pain and hardships of others. Now it is my turn to do what I can for other people who are going through difficult times and while easing their pain, help them to see that God is there for them too.

SURVIVOR'S GUIDE TO CHEMO 2.0

OVARIAN CANCER INFO

The following information was taken from The American Cancer Society (2018) website and the cancer-info-guide.com website:

Ovarian cancer is one of the most common types of cancers in women. According to research studies, ovarian cancer ranks fifth in cancer deaths among women. The chances of surviving ovarian cancer are better if the cancer is found early. But because the disease is difficult to detect in its early stage, only about 20% of ovarian cancers are found before tumor growth has spread into adjacent tissues and organs beyond the ovaries.

Stages:

Stage 1: The cancer is still contained within the ovary (or ovaries).

Stage 1A: Cancer has developed in one

ovary and the tumor is contained to the inside of the ovary. There is no cancer on the outer surface of the ovary. Laboratory examination of washings from the abdomen and pelvis did not find any cancer cells.

Stage 1B: Cancer has developed within both ovaries without any tumor on their outer surfaces. Laboratory examination of washings from the abdomen and pelvis did not find any cancer cells.

Stage 1C: The cancer is present in one or both ovaries and one or more of the following are present:

- Cancer on the outer surface of at least one of the ovaries.
- In the case of cystic tumors (fluid-filled tumors), the capsule (outer wall of the tumor) has ruptured.
- Laboratory examination found cancer cells in fluid or washings from the abdomen.

Stage 2: The cancer is in one or both

ovaries and has involved other organs (such as the uterus, fallopian tubes, bladder, the sigmoid colon, or the rectum) within the pelvis.

Stage 2A: The cancer has spread to or has actually invaded the uterus or the fallopian tubes, or both. Laboratory examination of washings from the abdomen did not find any cancer cells.

Stage 2B: The cancer has spread to other nearby pelvic organs such as the bladder, the sigmoid colon, or the rectum. Laboratory examination of washings from the abdomen did not find any cancer cells.

Stage 2C: The cancer has spread to pelvic organs as in stages 2A or 2B and laboratory examination of washings from the abdomen found evidence of cancer cells.

Stage 3: The cancer involves one or both ovaries, and one or both of the following are present: (1) cancer has spread beyond the pelvis to the lining of the abdomen; (2) cancer has spread to lymph nodes.

Stage 3A: During the staging operation, the

surgeon can see cancer involving the ovary or ovaries, but no cancer is grossly visible (can be seen without using a microscope) in the abdomen and the cancer has not spread to lymph nodes. However, when biopsies are checked under a microscope, tiny deposits of cancer are found in the lining of the upper abdomen.

Stage 3B: There is cancer in one or both ovaries, and deposits of cancer large enough for the surgeon to see, but smaller than 2 cm across, are present in the abdomen. Cancer has not spread to the lymph nodes.

Stage 3C: The cancer is in one or both ovaries, and one or both of the following are present:

- Cancer has spread to lymph nodes.
- Deposits of cancer larger than 2 cm across are seen in the abdomen.

Stage 4: This is the most advanced stage of ovarian cancer. The cancer is in one or both ovaries. Distant metastasis (spread of the cancer to the inside of the liver, the lungs, or other organs located outside of the peritoneal cavity) has occurred. Finding ovarian cancer cells in pleural fluid (from the cavity that surrounds the lungs) is also evidence of stage 4 disease ("Ovarian Cancer Stages," 2018).

SYMPTOMS

Ovarian cancer symptoms are nonspecific and mimic those of many other more common conditions, including digestive and bladder disorders. It isn't unusual for a woman with ovarian cancer to be diagnosed with another condition before finally learning she has cancer. The key seems to be persistent or worsening signs and symptoms. With most digestive disorders, symptoms tend to come and go, or they occur in certain situations or after eating certain foods. With ovarian cancer, there's typically little fluctuation where the symptoms are constant and gradually worsen. The most common symptoms are pain and swelling in the belly and gas. Other symptoms are diarrhea or constipation, or an upset stomach. Symptoms may include:

- Pressure or pain in the abdomen, pelvis, back or legs
- A swollen or bloated abdomen
- Nausea, indigestion, gas, constipation, or diarrhea
- Feeling very tired all of the time
- Shortness of breath
- Feeling the need to urinate often
- Unusual vaginal bleeding (heavy periods, or bleeding after menopause) ("Symptoms and Types," 2019).

NEW RESEARCH

New options are constantly being discovered
as researchers use genetic testing and genomic
sequencing to gain a better understanding of the
characteristics of ovarian cancer and how it can be
targeted with drugs. According to an article written
by Brielle Urciuoli (2018), some of the
advancements were reviewed by Ursula Matulonis,
M.D., chief of the Division of Gynecologic
Oncology at the Dana-Farber Cancer Institute in
Boston, on July 14th at the 2018 Ovarian Cancer
National Conference, in Washington D.C. In her
presentation which was sponsored by the Ovarian
Cancer Research Fund Alliance, Matulonis said,
"We know that ovarian cancer is not one cancer, but
trials in the past have really viewed it that way, so
advancements have been slow" (para. 1).

According to the American Cancer Society (2018), "research has led to better ways to detect high-risk genes and assess a woman's ovarian cancer risk. Studies suggest that many primary peritoneal cancers and some ovarian cancers (such as high-grade serous carcinomas) actually start in the fallopian tubes. According to this theory, the early changes of these cancers can start in the fallopian tubes. Cells from these very early fallopian tube cancers can become detached and then stick to the surface of the peritoneum or the ovaries. For reasons that are still not understood, these cancer cells may grow more rapidly in their new locations" (para. 4).

Detecting ovarian cancer early could have a great bearing on the cure rate. New ways of testing to screen women for ovarian cancer are being developed. "One method being tested is looking at the pattern of proteins in the blood (called proteomics) to find ovarian cancer early. For women who have an ovarian tumor, a test called OVA1 can measure the levels of 5 proteins in the blood. The levels of these proteins, when looked at together, are used to determine whether a woman's tumor should be considered low risk or high risk. If the tumor is labeled "low risk" based on this test, the woman is not likely to have cancer. If the tumor is considered "high risk," the woman is more likely to have a cancer and should see a specialist (a gynecologic oncologist). This test is NOT a screening test and it is NOT a test to decide if you should have surgery or not– it is meant for women who have an ovarian tumor where surgery has been decided but have not yet been referred to a gynecologic oncologist" (American Cancer Society, 2018, para. 9).

According to Cancer.net (2017), other targeted therapies include:

- "Immunotherapy. Immunotherapy is usually designed to boost the body's natural defenses to fight a cancer. It uses materials made either by the body or in a laboratory to bolster, target, or restore immune system function. Researchers are examining whether drugs called checkpoint inhibitors may boost the immune system's ability to destroy cancer cells. Drugs in this category target PD-1, PD-L1, and CTLA4. They have been shown to shrink tumors in other types of cancer, such as melanoma and some lung cancers, and have had some effectiveness in patients with ovarian/fallopian tube cancer.

- Cancer vaccines are another type of immunotherapy that researchers are testing for use against ovarian/fallopian tube cancer. Some approaches, called 'adoptive cell therapy,' use killer T cells from the immune system in an individual patient. Researchers take these cells and grow them in the laboratory, training them to attack certain targets, such as MUC 16 (CA-125), that are found on ovarian/fallopian tube cancer cells. Doctors then put the T cells back into the patient via an IV. This approach has been

tried with some early success in patients
with blood cancers.

- Hormone therapy. For treatment of
  recurrent or later-stage ovarian/fallopian
  tube cancer, tamoxifen, aromatase
  inhibitors, and enzalutamide (Xtandi), a
  blocker of the androgen receptor, are being
  studied.

- Gene therapy. A new area of research is
  discovering how damaged genes in
  ovarian/fallopian tube cancer cells can be
  corrected or replaced. Researchers are
  studying the use of specially designed
  viruses that carry normal genes into the core
  of cancer cells and then replace the defective
  genes with functional ones.

- Palliative care. Clinical trials are underway
  to find better ways of reducing symptoms
  and side effects of standard cancer
  treatments to improve a patient's comfort
  and quality of life" (para. 5).

AUTHORS NOTE

No financial gain was received by the author
from the Zimmer Center, New Hampshire Regional
Medical Center or any other company associated
with any brand name mentioned. This publication
is designed to provide accurate and authoritative
information in regard to the subject matter covered.
It is sold with the understanding that the author is
not engaged in rendering psychological, financial,
legal, or other professional services. If expert
assistance or counseling is needed, the services of a
competent professional should be sought.

REFERENCES

Ellis, A. (2019). Ovarian cancer research alliance
    FDA approved drugs for ovarian cancer.
    Retrieved from https://ocrahope.org/wp-
    content/uploads/2019/04/2019-SGO-report-
    final.pdf

Odunsi, K. (2018). How is immunotherapy
    changing the outlook for patients with
    ovarian cancer? Retrieved from
    https://www.cancerresearch.org/immunother
    apy/cancer-types/ovarian-cancer

Ovarian cancer guide: Symptoms and types. (2019).
    Retrieved from
    https://www.webmd.com/ovarian-
    cancer/guide/ovarian-cancer-symptoms-

types

Ovarian cancer stages. (2018). Retrieved from
    https://www.cancer.org/cancer/ovarian-
    cancer/detection-diagnosis-
    staging/staging.html?sitearea-cri&r=&bc=

Ovarian, fallopian tube, and peritoneal cancer:
    Latest research. (2017). Retrieved from
    https://www.cancer.net/cancer-
    types/ovarian-fallopian-tube-and-peritoneal-
    cancer/latest-research

Urciuoli, B. (2018). Exciting advancements
    underway in ovarian cancer. Retrieved from
    https://www.curetoday.com/conferences/ocn
    c-2018/exciting-advancements-underway-in-
    ovarian-cancer-

What's new in ovarian cancer research? (2018).
    Retrieved from
    https://www.cancer.org/cancer/ovarian-
    cancer/about/new-research.html

ABOUT THE AUTHOR

Deborah Waun is a Licensed Professional
Counselor, public speaker, and published author
with a Doctorate in Leadership and a Masters'
Degree in Psychology. She is an advocate for
women's rights and for helping women of all ages
to reach their greatest potential. Deborah became ill
in July and was diagnosed with ovarian cancer in
August of 2007. She spent close to a year
recovering from surgery and chemotherapy and was
considered in remission in July of 2008. During her
recovery, she wrote this book as a form of therapy
for herself and to help others going through similar
situations. She has been cancer-free since her
recovery.